The Garden Of Eaten

How To Eat And Lose 30 Pounds In 56 days

Rebecca Booker

The Garden Of Eaten: How To Eat And Lose 30 Pounds In 56 Days
Copyright © 2021 by Rebecca Booker

All rights reserved. No part of this book may be reproduced, distributed, or transmitted in any form or by any means, including photocopying, recording, or other electronic or mechanical methods, without the prior written permission of the author, except in the case of brief quotations embodied in critical reviews and certain other noncommercial uses permitted by copyright law. For permission requests, write to the author, addressed "Permissions Coordinator" at the address below.

Attention: Permissions Coordinator
P.O. Box 6676
Knoxville, TN 37914

MEDICAL DISCLAIMER:
This book may contain general information relating to healthy eating and positive impacts that some individuals with health issues have shared. Such information is provided for informational purposes only and is not meant to be a substitute for advice provided by a doctor or other qualified health care professionals. Individuals should not use the information in this book for health or weight loss without first consulting with their doctor and getting approval to do so.

*This book is dedicated to my mother
who has always supported my every endeavor.
Your belief in me is beyond measure,
and I am grateful to have a mother like you.*

*Mother of mine so wonderfully made
And hard to find; Mother of mine a
Love that lasts til' the end of time.*

—*Rebecca Booker*

TABLE OF CONTENTS

Acknowledgments i
Note From the Author v
Personal Information xi

Daily Meal Plan Menu: Week 1 1
Daily Meal Plan Menu: Week 2 8
Daily Meal Plan Menu: Week 3 15
Daily Meal Plan Menu: Week 4 22
Daily Meal Plan Menu: Week 5 29
Daily Meal Plan Menu: Week 6 36
Daily Meal Plan Menu: Week 7 43
Daily Meal Plan Menu: Week 8 50

Grocery List (Approved and Organic) 57
Approved Food Substitute List 59

ACKNOWLEDGMENTS

God – To my God, I thank you for giving me the vision to write this book. You are my inspiration for working with others to make this world that YOU created a better place. Without you and the journey that we have traveled together, there would be no book. For only *You* know the plans that you have for me. Plans for me to prosper and plans to give me a hope and a future. You are truly the way, the truth, and the life, and I will follow you to the ends of the earth.

Penny and Mr. Willie S. – Thanks to my parents who are the epitome of unconditional love. You have supported my endeavors throughout my entire life. Your love for me has been patient and kind, not self-seeking, and has not kept records of any of my shortcomings. Your love for me has never failed. It has given me a solid foundation to stand on and with that same love and dedication, I am inspired to share this book with the world.

Write My Wrongs Publishing Company – Thanks for taking a chance on me and bring my work to life so that my book will be available to others who are looking to eat healthy and lose weight.

Dr. LaVinia J. – Many thanks to you for being such an inspiration to me. Thanks for your willingness to listen and the encouragement to be excellent in my endeavors.

Dr. Stan B. – Much thanks to Dr. B, an extraordinary professor who once told me, "If you can write a sentence, then you can write a book. You were right! I thank you for all of your wisdom and encouragement throughout the years.

Pam E. (The Wellness Center) – Thank you for helping during one of the most difficult times in my life. I feel blessed to have met you, and I look forward to more conversations regarding the importance of good health!

Aliya & The Whole Foods Staff – Thank you for providing organic healthy food for families and investing in communities. The Whole

Foods Service has been excellent and extremely flexible throughout the Covid-19 pandemic. Shopping at your store has been a comforting experience during the pandemic. The staff at the Knoxville Whole Foods location is always so helpful and welcoming, and Whole Foods has become like a second home to me.

Barnes & Noble – Thank you for providing a place where people can meet and feel welcomed by the hospitality that your staff demonstrates each day. Your amazing selection of books, along with your staff, made the experience of two international students memorable.

Donna R. (Previous Director of The Cansler Family YMCA) – Thank you for believing in me and allowing me to have experienced a partnership with such an amazing organization.

Ed Financial – Thank you for the experience which helped me to get to this part of my journey. I am forever grateful.

Bobby M. – I would like to thank you Bobby for participating in *The Garden of Eaten* meal plan, and for believing in this book. I would also like to thank you for believing in me and encouraging me to write this book to help others achieve their weight loss goals.

Larry L. – Thanks for being such a wonderful friend and supporting me in all of my endeavors.

Deborah P. – Thanks to Mrs. Deborah for all of the love and support that you have given me through the years. You have been such a role model not only in excellence, but in the way that you serve the community. I hope to model your love and commitment in serving others.

Alan J. – You have influenced my life more than you could ever know. Thanks for being a wonderful mentor and great friend.

Umoja A. – Thank you for the love and support that you have given to me through the years and the wisdom that you always share during our conversations.

Paul M. – Much thanks to Paul, one of my dearest friends. You have always been supportive of me and encouraged me to continue writing. I am eternally grateful.

Atiba B. – Thank you for being supportive of my endeavors and the encouragement that you have given me over the years.

Carmen B. – Thank you for being such a good friend and all of the love, support, and encouragement that you have given me on my journey.

Andrea A. – Thank you for being there at a critical time in my life and building me up with your strength and prayers over my life. Glory to God!

Jarod A. – Thank you for being there at a critical time in my life and building me up with your strength and prayers for God to protect me and save my life. Glory to the Lord!

Ilene M. – Thank you for always being there and giving me support. I will always cherish your friendship!

Mike H. – Thanks for all of your encouragement and support through the years.

Brandi W. (U.S. Bank) – Thanks for all of your support during one of the most difficult times in my life. I will forever be grateful.

Halie (U.S. Bank) – Thank you for assisting me and offering support for my future endeavors!

Tonya W. (First-Sun Finance) – Thank you for assisting me at one of the most important time in my life. I am forever grateful.

Iris C. – Thank you for always showing support for my endeavors. You have been a great listener, but more importantly, a great friend.

Dewey R (Sr.) – Thank you for always believing in me. I appreciate all of the support that you have given me.

Pastor Dewey – Thank you for all of your support and discussions regarding health and communities in need of receiving better health options.

NOTE FROM THE AUTHOR

Thank you for joining me for breakfast and dinner! You, together with other individuals all over the world are my very special guest! I am delighted by your commitment to eating healthy and I am at your service during your quest for better health and weight loss. *The Garden of Eaten* menus are an effective, safe, and strategic way to eat healthy, lose weight, and reclaim your body! I applaud your commitment to a healthy eating lifestyle and there are a few things that I am willing to commit to you as well. I pledge to do the following: 1) Provide meal plan menus for two months; 2) Include information on how to eat and lose 30 pounds in 56 days; and 3) Provide a menu of foods that are organic and/or keto friendly including foods that research suggests can help strengthen the immune system, reduce inflammation, and improve overall health.

Very Important: Special Instructions Regarding Weight Loss
The meal plans are based on a low carb diet and they are also time-sensitive, meaning that individuals are encouraged to eat only TWICE a day and around the same time every day. This means that **NO SNACKS** should be eaten before, between, or after meals. It is recommended that the first meal is eaten at 12 noon. The second meal of the day (dinner) should be eaten either at 5pm or 6pm whichever fits your work schedule better. All dinner time meals must be eaten by 7pm with no exceptions, please. The times for eating meals are very important for weight loss results and if the times are not followed as mentioned above, then it could very much hinder your weight loss results. Another important thing that will need to be followed on this health journey is that you *MUST* make sure that you get enough **SLEEP** each night. This means having a goal to be in bed by 10pm or 11pm, if possible. The recommendation for sleep is at least 7-8 hours and the more sleep that you get, the better chance of getting phenomenal weight loss results!

In addition, it is suggested that ALL FOOD, SPICES, CONDIMENTS, and BEVERAGES should be ORGANIC. The majority of food on the menus are organic and/or paleo and keto friendly. The food that you cook must also be listed on the grocery list in the back of this book. Substitutes for food will be allowed, but they MUST be on the grocery list of approved foods. Individuals have experienced significant weight loss following a healthy eating lifestyle along with a time-sensitive breakfast and dinner meal. One testimonial comes from a 74-year-old man, named Bobby, who lost 32 pounds in 49 days when he prepared his meals from *The Garden of Eaten* meal plan menus. Not only did Bobby lose 32 pounds in a short time, but his blood pressure reduced and has consistently stayed in the normal range. Bobby had great results at his doctor visits and his doctor advised him to keep doing what he was doing because his medical results looked great!

This book was written for those of you who have struggled for years with weight issues. *The Garden of Eaten* was specifically created to assist individuals who are 50 or more pounds overweight. Individuals who are 20, 30, or 40 pounds overweight can also apply the same techniques in this book to lose weight, but I really wanted to reach out to individuals whose weight has caused long-term health issues or major insecurities of being seen in public, as well as individuals who might feel hopeless about ever being able to lose weight. Even if you are skeptical, I encourage you to try the meal plan menus and technique for yourself. How many diets are out there that allow you to eat healthy food that tastes great, lose weight (without exercise), and improve your overall health within 56 days? Ask yourself, is it worth your time to purchase this book, follow the daily food menus, and watch yourself lose 30 pounds in 56 days. *It is also recommended that you check with your doctor and maybe even request an allergy test and/or get your doctor's approval to eat the food included in the meal plan menus.* The *Garden of Eaten* is about eating the right foods, at the right time, and reclaiming your body!

Nutritional Facts

Losing weight is not just about eating fewer calories; it is also about eating healthy. Most diets focus on eating fewer calories. *The Garden of Eaten* focuses on the significance of eating healthy organic foods (low in sugar and carbs) that will not only assist the body in phenomenal weight loss, but also can help reduce inflammation and decrease risks for diseases, according to research. In the medical field, doctors are constantly telling patients to eat a healthy well balanced diet to reduce symptoms, relieve pain, and prevent certain illnesses from getting worse. However, how many people really know what foods are healthy and what foods are *not* healthy?

Many individuals have probably realized by now, that everything that is *said* to be healthy for the body is not always healthy and everything that is *said* to cause weight loss does not always work and often leads to gaining the weight back. As mentioned earlier, most individuals view weight loss as eating *fewer* calories and intensely working out. However, research has shown that eating a low carb diet along with eating *fewer* times a day is one of the most effective ways to not only lose weight, but it is also an excellent way to strengthen the immune system and improve overall health. It is important to **first** understand what is keeping you overweight or unhealthy. Did you know that every time you eat, it spikes the hormone called insulin? Whenever insulin is around, the body cannot lose weight because insulin is more dominant than the fat burning hormone known as the growth hormone, and this fat burning hormone cannot burn fat whenever insulin is around. Therefore, if a person eats several times throughout the day (including snacks), the fat burning hormone cannot burn fat and the chance of losing weight is slim. So, the questions that you are probably asking right now are **what** food can I eat, **when** can I eat it, and **how** can I eat and lose 30 pounds in 56 days? These are great questions and they are the main reason that this book of breakfast and dinner menus was written. The motivation for this book was derived from the hope that individuals like you would learn exactly *what* and *when* to eat in order to achieve phenomenal health and weight loss results. It is also recommended to consult with your doctor when changing your eating habits and preparing for a healthier lifestyle.

The Garden of Eaten outlines a health journey and the goal is not only to eat healthy and lose weight, but also to understand *why* you are eating the foods on the meal plans along with understanding the nutritional benefits of those food. As far as nutrition goes, let's start with the building blocks that are needed to keep the body running, known as v*itamins*! **Vitamins** build, defend, and maintain the body in using energy, healing wounds, and building muscle. We encourage others to learn about the importance of eating foods loaded with vitamins and minerals by talking with their doctors about vitamin enriched foods, and the nutrients that the body thrives on. The following information about vitamins and minerals may be of interest to you since they are in many of the foods included on the meal plan menus in this book.

VITAMIN A – helps with: acne, night blindness, dry eyes, and infections (sinus infections, ear infections, lung infections). Vitamin A gives support to the eye, skin, and the immune system. *Foods enriched with vitamin A:* kale, greens, carrots, and sweet potatoes.

VITAMIN B Complex (The nerve vitamins) – is a group of 8 water soluble vitamins which all play important roles in supporting different functions in your body since they directly impact your brain function, energy level, cell metabolism, and nerve health. Vitamin B complex also helps to gain recovery of nerve cells in the body. *Foods enriched with vitamin B complex:* dark leafy greens, eggs, beans, avocados, and meat.

VITAMIN C – enhances antibodies and it is a powerful anti-oxidant. Vitamin C can also help fight infection. *Foods enriched with vitamin C:* green leafy vegetables, bell peppers, sauerkraut, and berries.

VITAMIN D – protects against pathogens which are bacteria that harm your body. *Foods enriched with vitamin D:* egg yolks, salmon, tuna, sardines, oysters, cod liver, and shrimp.

VITAMIN E – prevents inflammation, helps heal burns, decreases the need for oxygen in the cell, and according to research, vitamin E increases collateral circulation (which is the re-routing of blood circulation around a blocked artery or vein via nearby minor vessels). Vitamin E can also help to prevent infection. Research suggests that vitamin E prevents nerve damage and can keep the blood from clotting. *Foods enriched with vitamin E:* salads, raw nuts, and raw seeds, leafy greens, avocados, egg yolks, almonds, kale, and Swiss chard.

VITAMIN K – According to research, if a person gets injured and does not have vitamin K1, they can literally bleed to death. Vitamin K2 keeps the calcium out of our blood vessels and prevents calcification. *Foods enriched with vitamin K:* leafy green vegetables, sauerkraut, egg yolks, chicken, beef, cheese, butter.

ZINC – is considered by some to be the most important trace mineral for the immune system. Zinc is a powerful antioxidant and a natural anti-Inflammatory. Research shows that zinc is supportive in reducing allergies and most people who have allergies are zinc deficient. High carb diets will deplete zinc. In addition, research shows that zinc is a natural anti-depressant. *Foods enriched with zinc:* beef, crabs, oysters.

Organic – According to research, organic means produce that is ground and processed without the use of chemical fertilizers or pesticides and no genetically modified organisms (GMO's). Organic food is a product of crops grown with soil that has not been treated for at least 3 years with any harmful substances that are prohibited and listed on the prohibited national list, such as synthetic pesticides, herbicides or synthetic fertilizers, which are harmful to crops and also harmful to the consumers who eat the crops. Organic food does not have any hormones added. *In order to be eligible for organic certification, land must be free of prohibited* *substances for 3 years and practices must be used that maintain or improve soil conditions and minimize erosion.* When choosing organic look for a label that reads USDA. The USDA label means 95% or more organic. If the label reads 100% USDA, then it means that the product is 100% organic.

Cholesterol – has often been viewed in a negative light. But it is also important to know a few things about cholesterol since some foods, such as eggs, are included in the meal plan menus. *Please research information on cholesterol so that doctors can provide updated information on how the body makes cholesterol, and its function in the body.* According to research, *cholesterol* acts as a coating for cell membrane and each cell in the body has cholesterol. Research also suggests that cholesterol is important and is necessary to make vitamin D. Cholesterol is also needed to make hormones including hormones for anti-inflammation. Cholesterol is involved in brain activity and research suggests that if you do not have enough *good* cholesterol, it can affect your memory. It is important to know that research has also shown that cholesterol is also needed to make bile, which helps to dissolve fat.

Personal Information

Beginning Date:

Name:

Date:

Weight:

Height:

Blood Pressure:

Medical Issues:

Weight Loss Goals: To Lose _____ in _____ months!

Previous weight loss programs that have been tried:

The Garden Of Eaten:
How To Eat And Lose 30 Pounds In 56 Days
By Rebecca Booker

Daily Meal Plan Menu: Week 1

Week 1/ Day 1

Your Breakfast/Brunch Menu for today is:
1) Sugar-Free Bacon - 2
2) Broccoli (Boil) - 1 Cup
3) Kale Salad (Stir-fry) - 1 Cup
4) Arugula Salad (Stir-fry) - 1 Cup
5) Waffle - 1/4 Serving
6) Water with Lemon - 8 oz.
7) Probiotics - Once A Day
8) Vitamin B Complex
Estimated Calories: 260
Estimated Carbs: 16.5
Estimated Sugar: 3.5
Blood Pressure (Optional):
Cooking Tip: Use coconut oil to stir-fry kale & arugula.

Your Dinner Menu for today is:
1) Chicken Breast - 1
2) Broccoli (Boil) - 1/2 Cup
3) Black Beans - 3 Tbsp
4) Slaw - 3 Tbsp
5) Water with Lemon - 8 oz.
Estimated Calories: 205
Estimated Carbs: 9.5
Estimated Sugar: 2.5 grams
Blood Pressure (Optional):
Cooking Tip: Cook chicken in air fryer or oven.

Go to: the-garden-of-eaten-book.com for cooking & coaching tips!

Daily Meal Plan Menu

Week 1/ Day 2

Your Breakfast/Brunch Menu for today is:
1) Sausage Patty - 1
2) Scrambled Egg - 2
3) Kale Salad (Stir-fry) - 1 Cup
4) Broccoli (Boil) - 1 Cup
5) Water with Lemon - 8 oz.
6) Probiotics - Once A Day
7) Vitamin B Complex
Estimated Calories: 260
Estimated Carbs: 9
Estimated Sugar: 1 gram
Blood Pressure (Optional):
Cooking Tip: Stir-fry kale with garlic salt is also an option.

Your Dinner Menu for today is:
1) Turkey Burger (No Bread) - 1
2) Kale Salad (Stir-fry) - 1 Cup
3) Arugula Salad (Stir-fry) - 1 Cup
4) Black Beans - 3 Tbsp
5) Slaw - 3 Tbsp
6) Water with Lemon - 8oz.
Estimated Calories: 280
Estimated Carbs: 12.5
Estimated Sugar: 2
Blood Pressure (Optional):
Cooking Tip: Use coconut oil to stir-fry kale & arugula.

Go to: the-garden-of-eaten-book.com for cooking & coaching tips!

Daily Meal Plan Menu

Week 1/ Day 3

Your Breakfast/Brunch Menu for today is:
1) Sausage Patty - 1
2) Scrambled Egg - 1
3) Asparagus (Boil) - 8 Stalks
4) Slaw - 3 Tbsp
5) Waffle - 1/4 Serving
6) Water with Lemon - 8 oz.
7) Probiotics - Once A Day
8) Vitamin B Complex
Estimated Calories: 410
Estimated Carbs: 9.5
Estimated Sugar: 4
Blood Pressure (Optional):
Cooking Tip: Mix slaw with avocado mayonnaise.

Your Dinner Menu for today is:
1) Kale Salad (Stir-fry) - 1 Cup
2) Arugula Salad (Stir-fry) - 1 Cup
3) Broccoli (Boil) - 1 Cup
4) Asparagus (Boil) - 8 Stalks
5) Slaw - 3 Tbsp
6) Water with Lemon - 8 oz
Estimated Calories: 150
Estimated Carbs: 15
Estimated Sugar: 2
Blood Pressure (Optional):
Cooking Tip: Use coconut oil to stir-fry kale & arugula.

Go to: the-garden-of-eaten-book.com for cooking & coaching tips!

Daily Meal Plan Menu

Week 1/ Day 4

Your Breakfast/Brunch Menu for today is:
1) Scrambled Eggs - 2
2) Broccoli (Boil) - 1/2 Cup
3) Kale Salad (Stir-fry) - 1 Cup
4) Arugula Salad (Stir-fry) - 1 Cup
5) Slaw - 3 Tbsp
6) Waffle - 1/4 Serving
7) Water with Lemon - 8oz.
8) Probiotics - Once A Day
9) Vitamin B Complex

Estimated Calories: 355
Estimated Carbs: 16.5
Estimated Sugar: 5
Blood Pressure (Optional):
Cooking Tip: Use coconut oil to stir-fry kale and arugula for 2 minutes.

Your Dinner Menu for today is:
1) Brussel Sprouts (Boil) - 5 Pieces
2) Broccoli (Boil) - 1/2 Cup
3) Black Beans - 3 Tbsp
4) Slaw - 3 Tbsp
5) Water with Lemon - 8 oz.

Estimated Calories: 115
Estimated Carbs: 11.5
Estimated Sugar: 2.5
Blood Pressure (Optional):
Cooking Tip: Mix slaw with avocado mayonnaise.

Go to: the-garden-of-eaten-book.com for cooking & coaching tips!

Daily Meal Plan Menu

Week 1/ Day 5

Your Breakfast/Brunch Menu for today is:
1) Scrambled Eggs - 2
2) Asparagus (Boil) - 8 Stalks
3) Avocado - 1 Whole
4) Broccoli (Boil) - 1 Cup
5) Water & Lemon - 8oz.
6) Probiotics - Once A Day
7) Vitamin B Complex
Estimated Calories: 300
Estimated Carbs: 8
Estimated Sugar: 1
Blood Pressure (Optional):
Cooking Tip: Boil asparagus and broccoli separately.

Your Dinner Menu for today is:
1) Buffalo Wings - 4 pieces (4 oz.)
2) Black Beans (Heat on stove) - 2 Tbsp
3) Kale (Stir-fry) - 1 Cup
4) Slaw - 3 Tbsp.
5) Water & Lemon - 8 oz.
Estimated Calories: 220
Estimated Carbs: 12.5
Estimated Sugar: 2
Blood Pressure (Optional):
Cooking Tip: Heat wings up and toss in buffalo wing sauce.

Go to: the-garden-of-eaten-book.com for cooking & coaching tips!

Daily Meal Plan Menu

Week 1/ Day 6

Your Breakfast/Brunch Menu for today is:
1) Boiled Eggs - 2
2) Asparagus (Boil) - 8 Stalks
3) Kale Salad (Stir-fry) - 1 Cup
4) Arugula Salad (Stir-fry) - 1 Cup
5) Slaw - 3 Tbsp
6) Water & Lemon - 8 oz.
7) Probiotics - Once A Day
8) Vitamin B Complex
Estimated Calories: 260
Estimated Carbs: 11
Estimated Sugar: 1
Blood Pressure (Optional):
Cooking Tip: Use coconut oil to stir-fry kale & arugula for 2 minutes.

Your Dinner Menu for today is:
1) Black Beans - 3 Tbsp.
2) Broccoli (Boil) - 1 Cup
3) Asparagus (Boil) - 8 Stalks
4) Brussel Sprouts (Boil) - 5 Pieces
5) Slaw - 3 Tbsp
6) Water & Lemon - 8 oz.
Estimated Calories: 160
Estimated Carbs: 10
Estimated Sugar: 2
Blood Pressure (Optional):
Cooking Tip: Boil each vegetable separately.

Go to: the-garden-of-eaten-book.com for cooking & coaching tips!

Daily Meal Plan Menu

Week 1/ Day 7

Your Breakfast/Brunch Menu for today is:
1) Sausage Patty - 1
2) Broccoli (Boil) - 1/2 Cup
3) Avocado - 1 Whole
4) Waffle - 1/4 Serving
5) Water & Lemon - 8 oz.
6) Probiotics - Once A Day
7) Vitamin B Complex
Estimated Calories: 285
Estimated Carbs: 9.5
Estimated Sugar: 3.5
Blood Pressure (Optional):
Cooking Tip: Cut avocado into pieces.

Your Dinner Menu for today is:
1) Asparagus (Boil) - 8 Stalks
2) Broccoli (Boil) - 1/2 Cup
3) Black Beans - 3 Tbsp
4) Slaw - 3 Tbsp
5) Water & Lemon - 8 oz.
Estimated Calories: 115
Estimated Carbs: 11.5
Estimated Sugar: 1.5
Blood Pressure (Optional):
Cooking Tip: Boil asparagus & broccoli separately.

Go to: the-garden-of-eaten-book.com for cooking & coaching tips!

The Garden Of Eaten:
How To Eat And Lose 30 Pounds In 56 Days
By Rebecca Booker

Daily Meal Plan Menu: Week 2

Week 2/ Day 8

Your Breakfast/Brunch Menu for today is:
1) Sugar-Free Bacon - 2
2) Broccoli (Boil) - 1/2 Cup
3) Arugula Salad (Stir-fry) - 1 Cup
4) Avocado Slices - 1 Whole
5) Waffle - 1/4 Serving
6) Water & Lemon - 8 oz.
7) Probiotics - Once A Day
8) Vitamin B Complex
Estimated Calories: 330
Estimated Carbs: 11.5
Estimated Sugar: 3.5
Blood Pressure (Optional):
Cooking Tip: Use coconut oil to stir-fry arugula

Your Dinner Menu for today is:
1) Baked Marinated Chicken Breast - 1 (4 oz)
2) Asparagus (Boil) - 1 Cup
3) Broccoli (Boil) - 1/2 Cup
4) Slaw - 3 Tbsp
5) Water & Lemon - 8 oz.
Estimated Calories: 180
Estimated Carbs: 6
Estimated Sugar: 1.5
Blood Pressure (Optional):
Cooking Tip: Use air fryer or oven to bake chicken breast.

Go to: the-garden-of-eaten-book.com for cooking & coaching tips!

Daily Meal Plan Menu

Week 2/ Day 9

Your Breakfast/Brunch Menu for today is:
1) Boiled Eggs - 2
2) Avocado Slices - 1
3) Broccoli (Stir-fry) - 1/2 Cup
4) Cauliflower (Stir-fry) - 1 Cup
5) Water & Lemon - 8 oz.
6) Probiotics - Once A Day
7) Vitamin B Complex
Estimated Calories: 285
Estimated Carbs: 6
Estimated Sugar: .5
Blood Pressure (Optional):
Cooking Tip: Use coconut oil & garlic salt to stir-fry broccoli & cauliflower.

Your Dinner Menu for today is:
1) Turkey Burger (No Bread) - 1
2) Black Beans - 3 Tbsp
3) Arugula Salad (Stir-fry) - 1 Cup
4) Slaw - 3 Tbsp
5) Water & Lemon - 8 oz.
Estimated Calories: 280
Estimated Carbs: 9.5
Estimated Sugar: 2
Blood Pressure (Optional):
Cooking Tip: Use coconut oil & garlic salt to stir-fry arugula.

Go to: the-garden-of-eaten-book.com for cooking & coaching tips!

Daily Meal Plan Menu

Week 2/ Day 10

Your Breakfast/Brunch Menu for today is:
1) Scrambled Eggs - 2
2) Broccoli (Boil) - 1/2 Cup
3) Asparagus (Boil) - 8 Stalks
4) Black Beans - 3 Tbsp
5) Slaw - 3 Tbsp
6) Waffle - 1/4 Serving
7) Water & Lemon - 8 oz.
8) Probiotics - Once A Day
9) Vitamin B Complex
Estimated Calories: 365
Estimated Carbs: 17
Estimated Sugar: 5.5
Blood Pressure (Optional):
Cooking Tip: Boil each vegetable separately.

Your Dinner Menu for today is:
1) Sausage Patty - 1
2) Broccoli (Boil) - 1/2 Cup
3) Asparagus (Boil) - 8 Stalks
4) Slaw - 3 Tbsp
5) Water & Lemon - 8 oz.
Estimated Calories: 245
Estimated Carbs: 4.5
Estimated Sugar: 1.5
Blood Pressure (Optional):
Cooking Tip: Boil broccoli and asparagus separately.

Go to: the-garden-of-eaten-book.com for cooking & coaching tips!

Daily Meal Plan Menu

Week 2/ Day 11

Your Breakfast/Brunch Menu for today is:
1) Sugar-Free Bacon - 2
2) Scrambled Egg - 1
3) Asparagus (Boil) - 8 Stalks
4) Avocado Slices - 1 Whole
5) Slaw - 3 Tbsp
6) Water & Lemon - 8 oz.
7) Probiotics - Once A Day
8) Vitamin B Complex
Estimated Calories: 290
Estimated Carbs: 6
Estimated Sugar: 1
Blood Pressure (Optional):
Cooking Tip: Mix slaw with avocado oil mayonnaise & 1 packet of organic raw sugar.

Your Dinner Menu for today is:
1) Scrambled Eggs - 2
2) Asparagus (Boil) - 8 Stalks
3) Arugula Salad (Stir-fry) - 1 Cup
4) Black Beans - 3 Tbsp
5) Sour Cream - 2 Tsp
6) Slaw - 3 Tbsp
7) Water & Lemon - 8 oz.
Estimated Calories: 300
Estimated Carbs: 13.5
Estimated Sugar: 2
Blood Pressure (Optional):
Cooking Tip: Mix black beans and sour cream.

Go to: the-garden-of-eaten-book.com for cooking & coaching tips!

Daily Meal Plan Menu

Week 2/ Day 12

Your Breakfast/Brunch Menu for today is:
1) Scrambled Egg - 1
2) Broccoli (Boil) - 1/2 Cup
3) Cauliflower (Boil) - 1 Cup
4) Slaw - 3 Tbsp
5) Waffle - 1/4 Serving
6) Water and Lemon - 8 oz.
7) Probiotics - Once A Day
8) Vitamin B Complex
Estimated Calories: 240
Estimated Carbs: 11.5
Estimated Sugar: 4.5
Blood Pressure (Optional):
Cooking Tip: Boil broccoli and cauliflower separately.

Your Dinner Menu for today is:
1) Turkey Burger (No Bread) - 1
2) Black Beans (Heat & Stir) - 3 Tbsp
3) Asparagus (Boil) - 8 Stalks
4) Arugula Salad (Stir-fry) - 1 Cup
5) Water and Lemon - 8 oz.
Estimated Calories: 290
Estimated Carbs: 9.5
Estimated Sugar: 1
Blood Pressure (Optional):
Cooking Tip: Garlic salt can be added to arugula for a great taste.

Go to: the-garden-of-eaten-book.com for cooking & coaching tips!

Daily Meal Plan Menu

Week 2/ Day 13

Your Breakfast/Brunch Menu for today is:
1) Homestyle Meatballs - 4
2) Scrambled Egg - 2
3) Broccoli (Boil) - 1/2 Cup
4) Brussel Sprouts (Boil) - 1/2 Cup
5) Water and Lemon - 8 oz.
6) Probiotics - Once A Day
7) Vitamin B Complex
Estimated Calories: 395
Estimated Carbs: 2.5
Estimated Sugar: .5
Blood Pressure (Optional):
Cooking Tip: Vegetables can be boiled or stir-fried.

Your Dinner Menu for today is:
1) Scrambled Eggs - 2
2) Broccoli (Boil) - 1/2 Cup
3) Asparagus (Boil) - 8 Stalks
4) Black Beans - 3 Tbsp
5) Slaw - 3 Tbsp
6) Water & Lemon - 8 oz.
Estimated Calories: 255
Estimated Carbs: 10
Estimated Sugar: 2.5
Blood Pressure (Optional):
Cooking Tip: Eggs can be scrambled or boiled.

Go to: the-garden-of-eaten-book.com for cooking & coaching tips!

Daily Meal Plan Menu

Week 2/ Day 14

Your Breakfast/Brunch Menu for today is:
1) Sugar-Free Bacon - 2
2) Broccoli (Boil) - 1/2 Cup
3) Slaw - 3 Tbsp
4) Waffle - 1/4 Serving
5) Water & Lemon - 8 oz.
6) Probiotics - Once A Day
7) Vitamin B Complex
Estimated Calories: 215
Estimated Carbs: 8
Estimated Sugar: 4.5
Blood Pressure (Optional):
Cooking Tip: Mix avocado mayonnaise with slaw.

Your Dinner Menu for today is:
1) Turkey Burger (No Bread) - 1
2) Asparagus (Boil) - 8 Stalks
3) Broccoli (Boil) - 1/2 Cup
4) Slaw - 3 Tbsp
5) Black Beans - 3 Tbsp
6) Sour Cream - 2 Tsp
7) Water & Lemon - 8 oz.
Estimated Calories: 295
Estimated Carbs: 13.5
Estimated Sugar: 2.5
Blood Pressure (Optional):
Cooking Tip: Mix slaw with avocado oil mayonnaise.

Go to: the-garden-of-eaten-book.com for cooking & coaching tips!

The Garden Of Eaten:
How To Eat And Lose 30 Pounds In 56 Days
By Rebecca Booker

Daily Meal Plan Menu: Week 3

Week 3/ Day 15

Your Breakfast/Brunch Menu for today is:
1) Wild Caught Cod (Bake) - 1
2) Scrambled Egg - 1
3) Kale (Stir-fry) - 1 Cup
4) Avocado - 1 Whole
5) Waffle - 1/4 Serving
6) Water & Lemon - 8 oz.
7) Probiotics - Once A Day
8) Vitamin B Complex
Estimated Calories: 400
Estimated Carbs: 12.5
Estimated Sugar: 3
Blood Pressure: (Optional)
Cooking Tip: Use coconut oil to stir-fry kale for 2 minutes.

Your Dinner Menu for today is:
1) Baked Marinated Chicken Breast - 1
2) Asparagus (Boil) - 8 Stalks
3) Broccoli (Boil) - 1/2 Cup
4) Slaw - 3 Tbsp
5) Water & Lemon - 8 oz.
Estimated Calories: 195
Estimated Carbs: 6
Estimated Sugar: 1.5
Blood Pressure (Optional):
Cooking Tip: Cook chicken breast in air fryer or oven at 425.

Go to: the-garden-of-eaten-book.com for cooking & coaching tips!

Daily Meal Plan Menu

Week 3/ Day 16

Your Breakfast/Brunch Menu for today is:
1) Boiled Eggs - 2
2) Broccoli (Boil) - 1/2 Cup
3) Avocado - 1 Whole
4) Slaw - 3 Tbsp
5) Waffle - 1/4 Serving
6) Water & Lemon - 8 oz.
7) Probiotics - Once A Day
8) Vitamin B Complex
Estimated Calories: 395
Estimated Carbs: 11.5
Estimated Sugar: 2.5
Blood Pressure (Optional):
Cooking Tip: Slice whole avocado into pieces.

Your Dinner Menu for today is:
1) 100% Grass-Fed Beef Burger (No Bread) - 1
2) Black Beans - 3 Tbsp
3) Asparagus (Boil) - 8 Stalks
4) Slaw - 3 Tbsp
5) Water & Lemon - 8 oz.
Estimated Calories: 320
Estimated Carbs: 9.5
Estimated Sugar: 2
Blood Pressure (Optional):
Cooking Tip: Mix avocado oil mayonnaise with slaw.

Go to: the-garden-of-eaten-book.com for cooking & coaching tips!

Daily Meal Plan Menu

Week 3/ Day 17

Your Breakfast/Brunch Menu for today is:
1) Broccoli (Boil) - 1 Cup
2) Asparagus (Boil) - 8 Stalks
3) Avocado - 1 Whole
4) Slaw - 3 Tbsp
5) Waffle - 1/4 Serving
5) Water & Lemon - 8 oz.
6) Probiotics - Once A Day
7) Vitamin B Complex
Estimated Calories: 300
Estimated Carbs: 15.5
Estimated Sugar: 2
Blood Pressure (Optional):
Cooking Tip: Boil broccoli & asparagus separately.

Your Dinner Menu for today is:
1) Baked Marinated Chicken Breast - 1
2) Broccoli (Boil) - 1/2 Cup
3) Brussel Sprouts (Boil) - 5
4) Slaw - 3 Tbsp
5) Water & Lemon - 8 oz.
Estimated Calories: 195
Estimated Carbs: 6
Estimated Sugar: 1.5
Blood Pressure (Optional):
Cooking Tip: Mix slaw with avocado mayonnaise.

Go to: the-garden-of-eaten-book.com for cooking & coaching tips!

Daily Meal Plan Menu

Week 3/ Day 18

Your Breakfast/Brunch Menu for today is:
1) Sugar-Free Bacon - 2
2) Scrambled Egg - 2
3) Broccoli (Boil) - 1/2 Cup
4) Asparagus (Boil) - 8 stalks
5) Water & Lemon - 8 oz.
6) Probiotics - Once A Day
7) Vitamin B Complex
Estimated Calories: 245
Estimated Carbs: 4
Estimated Sugar: 1
Blood Pressure (Optional):
Cooking Tip: Boil broccoli & asparagus separately.

Your Dinner Menu for today is:
1) Baked Marinated Chicken Breast - 1
2) Asparagus (Boil) - 8 Stalks
3) Broccoli (Boil) - 1/2 Cup
4) Brussel Sprouts (Boil) - 1/2 Cup
5) Slaw - 3 Tbsp
6) Water & Lemon - 8 oz.
Estimated Calories: 210
Estimated Carbs: 8
Estimated Sugar: 1.5
Blood Pressure (Optional):
Cooking Tip: (Boil vegetables separately).

Go to: the-garden-of-eaten-book.com for cooking & coaching tips!

Daily Meal Plan Menu

Week 3/ Day 19

Your Breakfast/Brunch Menu for today is:
1) Scrambled Egg - 2
2) Avocado - 1 Whole
3) Broccoli (Boil) - 1 Cup
4) Water & Lemon - 8 oz.
5) Probiotics - Once A Day
6) Vitamin B Complex
Estimated Calories: 270
Estimated Carbs: 6
Estimated Sugar: 1
Blood Pressure (Optional):
Cooking Tip: Slice whole avocado into pieces.

Your Dinner Menu for today is:
1) Sausage Patty - 1
2) Black Beans - 3 Tbsp
3) Asparagus (Boil) - 8 stalks
4) Brussel Sprouts (Boil) - 5 Pieces
5) Water & Lemon - 8 oz.
Estimated Calories: 200
Estimated Carbs: 9.5
Estimated Sugar: 1
Blood Pressure (Optional):
Cooking Tip: Boil vegetables separately.

Go to: the-garden-of-eaten-book.com for cooking & coaching tips!

Daily Meal Plan Menu

Week 3/ Day 20

Your Breakfast/Brunch Menu for today is:
1) Wild Caught Cod (Bake) - 1
2) Broccoli (Boil) - 1/2 Cup
3) Kale Salad (Stir-fry) - 1 Cups
4) Arugula Salad (Stir-fry) - 1 Cup
5) Avocado - 1 Whole
6) Water & Lemon - 8 oz.
7) Probiotics - Once A Day
8) Vitamin B Complex
Estimated Calories: 215
Estimated Carbs: 11
Estimated Sugar: 5
Blood Pressure (Optional):
Cooking Tip: Use coconut oil to stir-fry kale & arugula for 2 minutes.

Your Dinner Menu for today is:
1) Kale (Stir-fry) - 1 cup
2) Broccoli (Boil) - 1/2 Cup
3) Asparagus (Boil) - 8 Stalks
4) Slaw - 3 Tbsp
5) Avocado - 1 Whole
6) Water & Lemon - 8 oz.
Estimated Calories: 205
Estimated Carbs: 13
Estimated Sugar: 1.5
Blood Pressure (Optional):
Cooking Tip: Use coconut oil to stir-fry kale.

Go to: the-garden-of-eaten-book.com for cooking & coaching tips!

Daily Meal Plan Menu

Week 3/ Day 21

Your Breakfast/Brunch Menu for today is:
1) Sugar-Free Bacon - 2
2) Boiled Eggs - 2
3) Broccoli (Boil) - 1 Cup
4) Water & Lemon - 8 oz.
5) Probiotics - Once A Day
6) Vitamin B Complex
Estimated Calories: 230
Estimated Carbs: 4
Estimated Sugar: 1
Blood Pressure (Optional):
Cooking Tip: Eggs can also be scrambled or sunny side-up.

Your Dinner Menu for today is:
1) Home Style Meatballs - 4
2) Broccoli (Boil) - 1/2 Cup
3) Kale (Stir-fry) - 1 Cup
4) Slaw - 3 Tbsp
5) Water & Lemon - 8 oz.
Estimated Calories: 285
Estimated Carbs: 9
Estimated Sugar: 2
Blood Pressure (Optional):
Cooking Tip: Mix slaw with avocado mayonnaise.

Go to: the-garden-of-eaten-book.com for cooking & coaching tips!

The Garden Of Eaten:
How To Eat And Lose 30 Pounds In 56 Days
By Rebecca Booker

Daily Meal Plan Menu: Week 4

Week 4/ Day 22

Your Breakfast/Brunch Menu for today is:
1) Home Style Meatballs - 4
2) Broccoli (Boil) - 1 Cup
3) Cauliflower (Boil) - 1 Cup
4) Waffle - 1/4 Serving
5) Water with Lemon - 8 oz.
6) Probiotics - Once A Day
7) Vitamin B Complex
Estimated Calories: 365
Estimated Carbs: 11.5
Estimated Sugar: 4
Blood Pressure (Optional):
Cooking Tip: Boil broccoli & cauliflower separately.

Your Dinner Menu for today is:
1) Buffalo Wings - 4 (4oz.)
2) Black Beans - 3 Tbsp
3) Broccoli (Boil) - 1 Cup
4) Slaw - 3 Tbsp
5) Water with Lemon - 8 oz.
Estimated Calories: 290
Estimated Carbs: 11.5
Estimated Sugar: 3
Blood Pressure (Optional):
Cooking Tip: Bake wings & add mild or medium buffalo sauce).

Go to: the-garden-of-eaten-book.com for cooking & coaching tips!

Daily Meal Plan Menu

Week 4/ Day 23

Your Breakfast/Brunch Menu for today is:
1) Scrambled Eggs - 2
2) Avocado - 1 Whole
3) Broccoli (Boil) - 1 Cup
4) Water with Lemon - 8 oz.
5) Probiotics - Once A Day
6) Vitamin B Complex
Estimated Calories: 270
Estimated Carbs: 6
Estimated Sugar: 1
Blood Pressure (Optional):
Cooking Tip: Organic seasoning salt can be added to eggs.

Your Dinner Menu for today is:
1) Scrambled Eggs - 2
2) Black Beans - 3 Tbsp
3) Cauliflower (Boil) - 1/2 Cup
4) Slaw - 3 Tbsp
5) Water with Lemon - 8 oz.
Estimated Calories: 225
Estimated Carbs: 9.5
Estimated Sugar: 2
Blood Pressure (Optional):
Cooking Tip: Eggs can be boiled or scrambled.

Go to: the-garden-of-eaten-book.com for cooking & coaching tips!

Daily Meal Plan Menu

Week 4/ Day 24

Your Breakfast/Brunch Menu for today is:
1) Boiled Eggs - 2
2) Broccoli (Boil) - 1 Cup
3) Asparagus (Boil) - 8 Stalks
4) Slaw - 3 Tbsp
5) Water with Lemon - 8 oz.
6) Probiotics - Once A Day
7) Vitamin B Complex
Estimated Calories: 230
Estimated Carbs: 8
Estimated Sugar: 1
Blood Pressure (Optional):
Cooking Tip: Mix slaw with avocado mayonnaise.

Your Dinner Menu for today is:
1) Buffalo Wings - 4 (4oz.)
2) Broccoli (Boil) - 1 Cup
3) Black Beans - 3 Tbsp
4) Slaw - 3 Tbsp
5) Water with Lemon - 8 oz.
Estimated Calories: 290
Estimated Carbs: 11.5
Estimated Sugar: 3
Blood Pressure (Optional):
Cooking Tip: Bake wings & add mild or medium buffalo sauce.

Go to: the-garden-of-eaten-book.com for cooking & coaching tips!

Daily Meal Plan Menu

Week 4/ Day 25

Your Breakfast/Brunch Menu for today is:
1) Boiled Eggs - 2
2) Broccoli (Boil) - 1 Cup
3) Asparagus (Boil) - 8 Stalks
4) Waffle - 1/4 Serving
5) Water with Lemon - 8 oz.
6) Probiotics - Once A Day
7) Vitamin B Complex
Estimated Calories: 310
Estimated Carbs: 11.5
Estimated Sugar: 4
Blood Pressure (Optional):
Cooking Tip: Boil broccoli & asparagus separately.

Your Dinner Menu for today is:
1) 100% Grass-Fed Beef Burger (Fiesta Bowl) - 4oz.
2) Broccoli (Boil) - 1 Cup
3) Cauliflower (Boil) - 1/2 Cup
4) Black Beans - 3 Tbsp
5) Sour Cream - 2 Tsp
6) Grain-Free Tortilla Chips (with *Lime*) - 5
7) Water with Lemon - 8 oz.
Estimated Calories: 515
Estimated Carbs: 22.5
Estimated Sugar: 3
Blood Pressure (Optional):
Cooking Tip: Ground up beef burger & mix with black beans, sour cream & grain-free tortilla chips.

Go to: the-garden-of-eaten-book.com for cooking & coaching tips!

Daily Meal Plan Menu

Week 4/ Day 26

Your Breakfast/Brunch Menu for today is:
1) Sausage Patty - 1
2) Brussel Sprouts (Boil) - 5 pieces
3) Broccoli (Boil) - 1 Cup
4) Waffle - 1/4 Serving
5) Water with Lemon - 8 oz.
6) Probiotics - Once A Day
7) Vitamin B Complex
Estimated Calories: 340
Estimated Carbs: 11.5
Estimated Sugar: 4
Blood Pressure (Optional):
Cooking Tip: Boil broccoli and brussel sprouts separately.

Your Dinner Menu for today is:
1) Baked Marinated Chicken Breast - 1 (4 oz.)
2) Asparagus (Boil) - 8 Stalks
3) Broccoli (Boil) - 1/2 Cup
4) Kale Salad (Stir-fry) - 1 Cup
5) Arugula Salad (Stir-fry) - 1 Cup
6) Slaw - 3 Tbsp
7) Water with Lemon - 8 oz.
Estimated Calories: 255
Estimated Carbs: 13
Estimated Sugar: 1.5
Blood Pressure (Optional):
Cooking Tip: Use coconut oil to stir-fry kale & arugula for 2 minutes.

Go to: the-garden-of-eaten-book.com for cooking & coaching tips!

Daily Meal Plan Menu

Week 4/ Day 27

Your Breakfast/Brunch Menu for today is:
1) Scrambled Eggs - 2
2) Broccoli (Boil) - 1 Cup
3) Asparagus (Boil) - 8 Stalks
4) Cauliflower (Boil) - 1 Cup
5) Water with Lemon - 8 oz.
6) Probiotics - Once A Day
7) Vitamin B Complex
Estimated Calories: 215
Estimated Carbs: 6
Estimated Sugar: 1
Blood Pressure (Optional):
Cooking Tip: Boil broccoli & asparagus separately.

Your Dinner Menu for today is:
1) Baked Marinated Chicken Breast (4 oz) - 1
2) Cauliflower (Boil) - 1 Cup
3) Broccoli (Boil) - 1 Cup
4) Black Beans - 3 Tbsp
5) Water with Lemon - 8 oz.
Estimated Calories: 205
Estimated Carbs: 11.5
Estimated Sugar: 2
Blood Pressure (Optional):
Cooking Tip: Boil broccoli & cauliflower separately.

Go to: the-garden-of-eaten-book.com for cooking & coaching tips!

Daily Meal Plan Menu

Week 4/ Day 28

Your Breakfast/Brunch Menu for today is:
1) Scrambled Egg - 2
2) Broccoli (Boil) - 1/2 Cup
3) Kale (Stir-fry) - 1 Cup
4) Waffle - 1/4 Serving
5) Water with Lemon - 8 oz.
6) Probiotics - Once A Day
7) Vitamin B Complex
Estimated Calories: 295
Estimated Carbs: 12.5
Estimated Sugar: 3.5
Blood Pressure (Optional):
Cooking Tip: Use coconut oil to stir-fry kale for 2 minutes.

Your Dinner Menu for today is:
1) Sausage Patty - 1
2) Scrambled Eggs - 2
3) Broccoli (Boil) - 1 Cup
4) Slaw - 3 Tbsp
5) Water with Lemon - 8 oz.
Estimated Calories: 260
Estimated Carbs: 6
Estimated Sugar: 2
Blood Pressure (Optional):
Cooking Tip: Mix slaw with avocado mayonnaise.

Go to: the-garden-of-eaten-book.com for cooking & coaching tips!

The Garden Of Eaten:
How To Eat And Lose 30 Pounds In 56 Days
By Rebecca Booker

Daily Meal Plan Menu: Week 5

Week 5/ Day 29:

Your Breakfast/Brunch Menu for today is:
1) Sausage Patty - 1
2) Broccoli (Boil) - 1/2 Cup
3) Avocado - 1
4) Slaw - 3 Tbsp
5) Waffle - 1/4 Serving
6) Water & Lemon - 8 oz.
7) Probiotics - Once A Day
8) Vitamin B Complex
Estimated Calories: 375
Estimated Carbs: 11.5
Estimated Sugar: 4.5
Blood Pressure (Optional):
Cooking Tip: Mix slaw with avocado mayonnaise.

Your Dinner Menu for today is:
1) Wild Caught Cod (Bake) - 1
2) Broccoli (Boil) - 1 Cup
3) Kale Salad (Stir-fry) - 1 Cup
4) Slaw - 3 Tbsp
5) Water & Lemon - 8 oz.
Estimated Calories: 200
Estimated Carbs: 11
Estimated Sugar: 2
Blood Pressure (Optional):
Cooking Tip: Mix slaw with avocado mayonnaise.

Go to: the-garden-of-eaten-book.com for cooking & coaching tips!

Daily Meal Plan Menu

Week 5/ Day 30

Your Breakfast/Brunch Menu for today is:
1) Scrambled Eggs - 2
2) Brussel Sprouts (Boil) - 5 pieces
3) Asparagus (Boil) - 8 Stalks
4) Broccoli (Boil) - 1 Cup
5) Water & Lemon - 8 oz.
6) Probiotics - Once A Day
7) Vitamin B Complex
Estimated Calories: 230
Estimated Carbs: 8
Estimated Sugar: 1
Blood Pressure (Optional):
Cooking Tip: Boil brussel sprouts, broccoli & asparagus separately.

Your Dinner Menu for today is:
1) Turkey Burger (No Bread) - 1
2) Kale Salad (Stir-fry) - 1 Cup
3) Arugula Salad (Stir-fry) - 1Cup
4) Slaw - 3 Tbsp
5) Water & Lemon - 8 oz.
Estimated Calories: 240
Estimated Carbs: 9
Estimated Sugar: 1
Blood Pressure (Optional):
Cooking Tip: Use coconut oil to stir-fry kale & arugula for 2 minutes.

Go to: the-garden-of-eaten-book.com for cooking & coaching tips!

Daily Meal Plan Menu

Week 5/ Day 31

Your Breakfast/Brunch Menu for today is:
1) Boiled Eggs - 2
2) Avocado -1
3) Broccoli (Boil) - 1 Cup
4) Waffle - 1/4 Serving
5) Water & Lemon - 8 oz.
6) Probiotics - Once A Day
7) Vitamin B Complex
Estimated Calories: 380
Estimated Carbs: 11.5
Estimated Sugar: 4
Blood Pressure (Optional):
Cooking Tip: Slice whole avocado into pieces.

Your Dinner Menu for today is:
1) Sugar-Free Bacon - 2
2) Black Beans - 3 Tbsp
3) Grain-Free Tortilla Chips (with *Lime*) - 5 pieces
4) Organic Sour Cream - 2 Tsp
5) Slaw - 3 Tbsp
6) Water & Lemon - 8 oz.
Estimated Calories: 350
Estimated Carbs: 18.5
Estimated Sugar: 3
Blood Pressure (Optional):
Cooking Tip: Mix black beans with sour cream and grain-free tortilla chips.

Go to: the-garden-of-eaten-book.com for cooking & coaching tips!

Daily Meal Plan Menu

Week 5/ Day 32

Your Breakfast/Brunch Menu for today is:
1) Home Style Meatballs - 4
2) Scrambled Eggs - 2
3) Avocado – 1 Whole
4) Waffle - 1/4 Serving
5) Water & Lemon - 8 oz.
6) Probiotics - Once A Day
7) Vitamin B Complex
Estimated Calories: 580
Estimated Carbs: 7.5
Estimated Sugar: 3
Blood Pressure (Optional):
Cooking Tip: Slice whole avocado into pieces.

Your Dinner Menu for today is:
1) Wild Caught Cod (Bake) - 1
2) Broccoli (Boil) - 1/2 Cup
3) Kale Salad (Stir-fry) - 1 Cup
4) Arugula Greens (Stir-fry) - 1 Cup
5) Water & Lemon - 8 oz.
Estimated Calories: 195
Estimated Carbs: 9
Estimated Sugar: .5
Blood Pressure (Optional):
Cooking Tip: Use coconut oil to stir-fry kale & arugula for 2 minutes.

Go to: the-garden-of-eaten-book.com for cooking & coaching tips!

Daily Meal Plan Menu

Week 5/ Day 33

Your Breakfast/Brunch Menu for today is:
1) Turkey Burger (No Bread) - 1
2) Scrambled Eggs - 2
3) Kale Salad (Stir-fry) - 1 Cup
4) Arugula Salad (Stir-fry) - 1 Cup
5) Water & Lemon - 8 oz.
6) Probiotics - Once A Day
7) Vitamin B Complex
Estimated Calories: 350
Estimated Carbs: 7
Estimated Sugar: 0
Blood Pressure (Optional):
Cooking Tip: Use coconut oil to stir-fry kale & arugula for 2 minutes.

Your Dinner Menu for today is:
1) Asparagus (Boil) - 8 Stalks
2) Broccoli (Boil) - 1/2 Cup
3) Kale Salad (Stir-fry) - 1 Cup
4) Black Beans - 3 Tbsp
5) Slaw - 3 Tbsp
6) Water & Lemon - 8 oz.
Estimated Calories: 145
Estimated Carbs: 14.5
Estimated Sugar: 2.5
Estimated Blood Pressure (Optional):
Cooking Tip: Boil broccoli & asparagus separately.

Go to: the-garden-of-eaten-book.com for cooking & coaching tips!

Daily Meal Plan Menu

Week 5/ Day 34

Your Breakfast/Brunch Menu for today is:
1) Sugar-Free Bacon - 2
2) Broccoli (Boil) - 1/2 Cup
3) Cauliflower (Boil) - 1/2 Cup
4) Waffles - 1/4 Serving
5) Water & Lemon - 8 oz.
6) Probiotics - Once A Day
7) Vitamin B Complex
Estimated Calories: 260
Estimated Carbs: 9.5
Estimated Sugar: 3.5
Blood Pressure (Optional):
Cooking Tip: Boil broccoli & cauliflower separately.

Your Dinner Menu for today is:
1) Baked Marinated Chicken Breast - 1
2) Asparagus (Boil) - 8 Stalks
3) Kale Salad (Stir-fry) - 1 Cup
4) Arugula Salad (Stir-fry) - 1 Cup
5) Slaw - 3 Tbsp
6) Water & Lemon - 8 oz.
Estimated Calories: 240
Estimated Carbs: 11
Estimated Sugar: 1
Blood Pressure (Optional):
Cooking Tip: Stir-fry kale & arugula with coconut oil.

Go to: the-garden-of-eaten-book.com for cooking & coaching tips!

Daily Meal Plan Menu

Week 5/ Day 35

Your Breakfast/Brunch Menu for today is:
1) Home Style Meatballs - 4
2) Scrambled Egg - 2
3) Broccoli (Boil) - 1 Cup
4) Waffle - 1/4 Serving
5) Water & Lemon - 8 oz.
6) Probiotics - Once A Day
7) Vitamin B Complex
6**Estimated Calories:** 490
Estimated Carbs: 9.5
Estimated Sugar: 4
Blood Pressure: (Optional)
Cooking Tip: Mozzarella cheese can be sprinkled on broccoli (1 Tsp.)

Your Dinner Menu for today is:
1) Turkey Burger (No Bread) - 1
2) Black Beans - 3 Tbsp
3) Kale Salad (Stir-fry) - 1 Cup
4) Arugula Salad (Stir-fry) - 1 Cup
5) Water & Lemon - 8 oz.
Estimated Calories: 250
Estimated Carbs: 9.5
Estimated Sugar: 1
Blood Pressure (Optional):
Cooking Tip: Use coconut oil to stir-fry kale & arugula salad.

Go to: the-garden-of-eaten-book.com for cooking & coaching tips!

The Garden Of Eaten:
How To Eat And Lose 30 Pounds In 56 Days
By Rebecca Booker

Daily Meal Plan Menu: Week 6

Week 6/ Day 36

Your Breakfast/Brunch Menu for today is:
1) Sausage Patty -1
2) Broccoli (Boil) - 1 Cup
3) Avocado - 1 Whole
4) Slaw - 3 Tbsp
5) Water & Lemon - 8 oz.
6) Probiotics - Once A Day
7) Vitamin B Complex
Estimated Calories: 330
Estimated Carbs: 8
Estimated Sugar: 2
Blood Pressure (Optional):
Cooking Tip: Slice whole avocado into pieces.

Your Dinner Menu for today is:
1) Wild Caught Cod (Bake) - 1
2) Broccoli (Boil) - 1 Cup
3) Kale Salad (Stir-fry) - 1 Cup
4) Slaw - 3 Tbsp
5) Water & Lemon - 8 oz.
Estimated Calories: 180
Estimated Carbs: 11
Estimated Sugar: 2
Blood Pressure (Optional):
Cooking Tip: Mix slaw with avocado mayonnaise.

Go to: the-garden-of-eaten-book.com for cooking & coaching tips!

Daily Meal Plan Menu

Week 6/ Day 37

Your Breakfast/Brunch Menu for today is:
1) Scrambled Eggs - 2
2) Avocado - 1 Whole
3) Broccoli (Boil) - 1 Cup
4) Cauliflower (Boil) - 1/2 Cup
5) Water & Lemon - 8 oz.
6) Probiotics - Once A Day
7) Vitamin B Complex
Estimated Calories: 285
Estimated Carbs: 8
Estimated Sugar: 1
Blood Pressure (Optional):
Cooking Tip: Cut whole avocado into pieces.

Your Dinner Menu for today is:
1) Baked Marinated Chicken Breast - 4 oz
2) Kale Salad (Stir-fry) - 1 Cup
3) Arugula Salad (Stir-fry) - 1 Cup
4) Asparagus (Boil) - 8 Stalks
5) Slaw - 3 Tbsp
6) Water & Lemon - 8 oz.
Estimated Calories: 240
Estimated Carbs: 11
Estimated Sugar: 1
Blood Pressure (Optional):
Cooking Tip: Use coconut oil to stir-fry kale & arugula for 2 minutes.

Go to: the-garden-of-eaten-book.com for cooking & coaching tips!

Daily Meal Plan Menu

Week 6/ Day 38

Your Breakfast/Brunch Menu for today is:
1) Sugar-Free Bacon - 2
2) Cauliflower (Boil) - 1/2 Cup
3) Broccoli (Boil) - 1 Cup
4) Waffle - 1/4 - Serving
5) Water & Lemon - 8 oz.
6) Probiotics - Once A Day
7) Vitamin B Complex
Estimated Calories: 215
Estimated Carbs: 11.5
Estimated Sugar: 4
Blood Pressure (Optional):
Cooking Tip: Turkey bacon can be used as an alternative.

Your Dinner Menu for today is:
1) Wild Caught Cod (Bake) - 1
2) Broccoli (Boil) - 1 Cup
3) Asparagus (Boil) - 8 Stalks
4) Slaw - 3 Tbsp
5) Water & Lemon - 8 oz.
Estimated Calories: 180
Estimated Carbs: 8
Estimated Sugar: 2
Blood Pressure (Optional):
Cooking Tip: Mix slaw with avocado mayonnaise.

Go to: the-garden-of-eaten-book.com for cooking & coaching tips!

Daily Meal Plan Menu

Week 6/ Day 39

Your Breakfast/Brunch Menu for today is:
1) Sugar-Free Bacon - 2
2) Broccoli (Boil) - 1/2 Cup
3) Avocado - 1 Whole
4) Asparagus (Boil) - 8 stalks
5) Waffle - 1/4 Serving
6) Water & Lemon - 8 oz.
7) Probiotics - Once A Day
8) Vitamin B Complex
Estimated Calories: 315
Estimated Carbs: 11.5
Estimated Sugar: 3.5
Blood Pressure (Optional):
Cooking Tip: Boil broccoli & asparagus separately.

Your Dinner Menu for today is:
1) Black Beans - 3 Tbsp
2) Slaw - 3 Tbsp
3) Kale Salad (Stir-fry) - 1 Cup
4) Arugula Salad (Stir-fry) - 1 Cup
5) Avocados - 1 Whole
6) Water & Lemon - 8 oz.
Estimated Calories: 230
Estimated Carbs: 17.5
Estimated Sugar: 2
Blood Pressure (Optional):
Cooking Tip: Use coconut oil to stir-fry kale & arugula for 2 minutes.

Go to: the-garden-of-eaten-book.com for cooking & coaching tips!

Daily Meal Plan Menu

Week 6/ Day 40

Your Breakfast/Brunch Menu for today is:
1) Sausage Patty - 1
2) Scrambled Eggs - 2
3) Asparagus (Boil) - 8 Stalks
4) Slaw - 3 Tbsp.
5) Water & Lemon - 8 oz.
6) Probiotics - Once A Day
7) Vitamin B Complex
Estimated Calories: 320
Estimated Carbs: 4
Estimated Sugar: 1
Blood Pressure (Optional):
Cooking Tip: Eggs can be scrambled or boiled.

Your Dinner Menu for today is:
1) Turkey Burger (No Bread) - 1
2) Black Beans - 3 Tbsp.
3 Asparagus (Boil) - 8 Stalks
4) Grain-Free Tortilla Chips - 5
5) Sour Cream - 2 Tbsp
6) Water & Lemon - 8 oz.
Estimated Calories: 380
Estimated Carbs: 18.5
Estimated Sugar: 2
Blood Pressure (Optional):
Cooking Tip: Mix black beans with sour cream & grain-free tortilla chips.

Go to: the-garden-of-eaten-book.com for cooking & coaching tips!

Daily Meal Plan Menu

Week 6/ Day 41

Your Breakfast/Brunch Menu for today is:
1) Wild Caught Cod (Bake) - 1
2) Broccoli (Boil) - 1/2 Cup
3) Avocado - 1 Whole
4) Waffle - 1/4 Serving
5) Water & Lemon - 8 oz.
6) Probiotics - Once A Day
7) Vitamin B Complex
Estimated Calories: 315
Estimated Carbs: 9.5
Estimated Sugar: 4
Blood Pressure (Optional):
Cooking Tip: Cut whole avocado into slices.

Your Dinner Menu for today is:
1) 100% Grass-Fed Burger (No Bread) - 4oz.
2) Black Beans - 3 Tbsp
3) Asparagus (Boil) - 8 Stalks
4) Broccoli (Boil) - 1 Cup
5) Sour Cream - 2 Tbsp
6) Water & Lemon - 8 oz.
Estimated Calories: 350
Estimated Carbs: 13.5
Estimated Sugar: 2
Blood Pressure (Optional):
Cooking Tip: Mix cooked ground beef patty and black beans with sour cream.

Go to: the-garden-of-eaten-book.com for cooking & coaching tips!

Daily Meal Plan Menu

Week 6/ Day 42

Your Breakfast/Brunch Menu for today is:
1) Scrambled Eggs - 2
2) Broccoli (Boil) - 1 Cup
3) Asparagus (Boil) - 8 Stalks
4) Cauliflower (Boil) - 1/2 Cup
4) Water & Lemon - 8 oz.
5) Probiotics - Once A Day
6) Vitamin B Complex
Estimated Calories: 215
Estimated Carbs: 8
Estimated Sugar: 1
Blood Pressure (Optional):
Cooking Tip: Boil broccoli & cauliflower separately.

Your Dinner Menu for today is:
1) Sausage Patty - 1
2) Broccoli - 1/2 Cup
3) Kale Salad (Stir-fry) - 1 Cup
4) Arugula Salad (Stir-fry) - 1 Cup
5) Slaw - 3 Tbsp
6) Water & Lemon - 8oz.
Estimated Calories: 165
Estimated Carbs: 11
Estimated Sugar: 2.5
Blood Pressure (Optional):
Cooking Tip: Use coconut oil to stir-fry kale & arugula for 2 minutes.

Go to: the-garden-of-eaten-book.com for cooking & coaching tips!

The Garden Of Eaten:
How To Eat And Lose 30 Pounds In 56 Days
By Rebecca Booker

Daily Meal Plan Menu: Week 7

Week 7/ Day 43

Your Breakfast/Brunch Menu for today is:
1) Turkey Burger (No Bread) - 1
2) Scrambled Eggs - 2
3) Asparagus (Boil) - 8 Stalks
4) Waffle - 1/4 Serving
5) Water & Lemon - 8 oz.
6) Probiotics - Once A Day
7) Vitamin B Complex
Estimated Calories: 430
Estimated Carbs: 7.5
Estimated Sugar: 3
Blood Pressure (Optional):
Cooking Tip: Eggs can also be boiled or cooked sunny-side up.

Your Dinner Menu for today is:
1) Sugar-Free Bacon - 2
2) Broccoli (Boil) - 1/2 Cup
3) Black Beans - 3 Tbsp
4) Slaw - 3 Tbsp
5) Water & Lemon - 8 oz.
Estimated Calories: 205
Estimated Carbs: 9.5
Estimated Sugar: 2.5
Blood Pressure (Optional):
Cooking Tip: Mix slaw with avocado oil mayonnaise.

Go to: the-garden-of-eaten-book.com for cooking & coaching tips!

Daily Meal Plan Menu

Week 7/ Day 44

Your Breakfast/Brunch Menu for today is:
1) Boiled Eggs - 2
2) Broccoli (Boil) - 1/2 Cup
3) Cauliflower (Boil) - 1/2 Cup
4) Kale Salad (Stir-fry) - 1 Cup
5) Water & Lemon - 8 oz.
6) Probiotics - Once A Day
7) Vitamin B Complex
Estimated Calories: 200
Estimated Carbs: 9
Estimated Sugar: 1
Blood Pressure (Optional):
Cooking Tip: Use coconut oil to stir-fry kale for 2 minutes.

Your Dinner Menu for today is:
1) Turkey Burger - 1
2) Slaw - 3 Tbsp
3) Broccoli (Boil) - 1/2 Cup
4) Asparagus (Boil) - 8 Stalks
5) Waffle - 3 Tbsp
6) Water & Lemon - 8 oz.
Estimated Calories: 335
Estimated Carbs: 11.5
Estimated Sugar: 5
Blood Pressure (Optional):
Cooking Tip: Boil broccoli & asparagus separately.

Go to: the-garden-of-eaten-book.com for cooking & coaching tips!

Daily Meal Plan Menu

Week 7/ Day 45

Your Breakfast/Brunch Menu for today is:
1) Scrambled Eggs - 2
2) Avocado - 1 Whole
3) Broccoli (Boil) - 1/2 Cup
4) Cauliflower (Boil) - 1/2 Cup
5) Waffle - 1/4 Serving
6) Water & Lemon - 8 oz.
7) Probiotics - Once A Day
8) Vitamin B Complex
Estimated Calories: 380
Estimated Carbs: 11.5
Estimated Sugar: 4
Blood Pressure (Optional):
Cooking Tip: Eggs can be boiled or sunny-side up.

Your Dinner Menu for today is:
1) Sugar-Free Bacon - 2
2) Broccoli (Boiled) - 1/2 Cup
3) Cauliflower (Boiled) - 1/2 Cup
4) Arugula Salad (Stir-fry) - 1 Cup
5) Grain-Free Tortilla Chips (with *Lime*) - 5
6) Black Beans - 2 Tbsp
7) Sour Cream - 2 Tsp
8) Water & Lemon - 8 oz.
Estimated Calories: 335
Estimated Carbs: 22.5
Estimated Sugar: 2.5
Blood Pressure (Optional):
Cooking Tip: Mix black beans and sour cream with grain-free tortilla chips.

Go to: the-garden-of-eaten-book.com for cooking & coaching tips!

Daily Meal Plan Menu

Week 7/ Day 46

Your Breakfast/Brunch Menu for today is:
1) Sugar-Free Bacon - 2
2) Scrambled Egg - 2
3) Brussel Sprouts (Boil) - 5 Pieces
4) Asparagus (Boil) - 8 Stalks
5) Water & Lemon - 8 oz.
6) Probiotics - Once A Day
7) Vitamin B Complex
Estimated Calories: 260
Estimated Carbs: 4
Estimated Sugar: 0
Blood Pressure (Optional):
Cooking Tip: Eggs can also be boiled or sunny-side up or boiled.

Your Dinner Menu for today is:
1) Home Style Meatballs (Fiesta Bowl) - 4
2) Broccoli (Boil) - 1/2 Cup
3) Black Beans - 3 Tbsp
4) Grain-Free Tortilla Chips (with *Lime*) - 5
5) Sour Cream - 2 Tsp
6) Water & Lemon - 8 oz.
Estimated Calories: 435
Estimated Carbs: 18.5
Estimated Sugar: 3
Blood Pressure (Optional):
Cooking Tip: (Mix cooked home style meatballs with, black beans, sour cream, & grain-free tortilla chips).

Go to: the-garden-of-eaten-book.com for cooking & coaching tips!

Daily Meal Plan Menu

Week 7/ Day 47

Your Breakfast/Brunch Menu for today is:
1) Turkey Burger (No Bread) - 1
2) Scrambled Eggs - 2
3) Asparagus (Boil) - 8 Stalks
4) Broccoli (Boil) - 1/2 Cup
5) Slaw - 3 Tbsp
6) Water & Lemon - 8 oz.
7) Probiotics - Once A Day
8) Vitamin B Complex
Estimated Calories: 365
Estimated Carbs: 6
Estimated Sugar: 1.5
Blood Pressure (Optional):
Cooking Tip: Boil asparagus and broccoli separately.

Your Dinner Menu for today is:
1) Home Style Meatballs - 4
2) Broccoli (Boil) - 1 Cup
3) Cauliflower (Boil) - 1 Cup
4) Slaw - 3 Tbsp
5) Water & Lemon - 8 oz.
Estimated Calories: 285
Estimated Carbs: 8
Estimated Sugar: 2
Blood Pressure (Optional):
Cooking Tip: Mix slaw with avocado oil mayonnaise.

Go to: the-garden-of-eaten-book.com for cooking & coaching tips!

Daily Meal Plan Menu

Week 7/ Day 48

Your Breakfast/Brunch Menu for today is:
1) Sausage Patty - 1
2) Boiled Eggs - 2
3) Broccoli (Boil) - 1 Cup
4) Waffle - 1/4 Serving
5) Water & Lemon - 8 oz.
6) Probiotics - Once A Day
7) Vitamin B Complex
Estimated Calories: 450
Estimated Carbs: 9.5
Estimated Sugar: 4
Blood Pressure (Optional):
Cooking Tip: Eggs can also be cooked sunny-side up.

Your Dinner Menu for today is:
1) Baked Marinated Chicken Breast
2) Broccoli (Stir-fry) - 1/2 Cup
3) Kale Salad (Stir-fry) - 1 Cup
4) Slaw - 3 Tbsp
5) Water & Lemon - 8 oz.
Estimated Calories: 195
Estimated Carbs: 9
Estimated Sugar: 1.5
Blood Pressure (Optional):
Cooking Tip: Use coconut oil to stir-fry kale & broccoli for 2 minutes.

Go to: the-garden-of-eaten-book.com for cooking & coaching tips!

Daily Meal Plan Menu

Week 7/ Day 49

Your Breakfast/Brunch Menu for today is:
1) Turkey Burger - 1
2) Kale Salad (Stir-fry) - 1 Cup
3) Arugula Salad (Stir-fry) - 1 Cup
4) Black Beans - 3 Tbsp
5) Slaw - 3 Tbsp
6) Water & Lemon - 8 oz.
7) Probiotics - Once A Day
8) Vitamin B Complex
Estimated Calories: 280
Estimated Carbs: 14.5
Estimated Sugar: 2
Blood Pressure (Optional):
Cooking Tip: Use coconut oil to stir-fry kale & arugula for 2 minutes.

Your Dinner Menu for today is:
1) Scrambled Eggs - 2
2) Black Beans - 2 Tbsp
3) Broccoli (Boil) - 1/2 Cup
4) Asparagus (Boil) - 8 Stalks
5) Slaw - 3 Tbsp
6) Water & Lemon - 8 oz.
Estimated Calories: 255
Estimated Carbs: 11.5
Estimated Sugar: 2.5
Blood Pressure (Optional):
Cooking Tip: Boil broccoli & asparagus separately.

Go to: the-garden-of-eaten-book.com for cooking & coaching tips!

The Garden Of Eaten:
How To Eat And Lose 30 Pounds In 56 Days
By Rebecca Booker

Daily Meal Plan Menu: Week 8

Week 8/ Day 50

Your Breakfast/Brunch Menu for today is:
1) Turkey Burger - 1
2) Broccoli (Boil) - 1/2 Cup
3) Cauliflower (Boil) - 1 Cup
4) Waffle - 1/4 Serving
5) Slaw - 3 Tbsp
6) Water & Lemon - 8 oz.
7) Probiotics - Once A Day
8) Vitamin B Complex
Estimated Calories: 320
Estimated Carbs: 11.5
Estimated Sugar: 4.5
Blood Pressure (Optional):
Cooking Tip: Mix slaw with avocado mayonnaise.

Your Dinner Menu for today is:
1) Sausage Patty - 1
2) Asparagus (Boil) - 8 Stalks
3) Broccoli (Boil) - 1 Cup
4) Slaw - 3 Tbsp
5) Water & Lemon - 8 oz.
Estimated Calories: 150
Estimated Carbs: 8
Estimated Sugar: 2
Blood Pressure (Optional):
Cooking Tip: Boil broccoli & asparagus separately.

Go to: the-garden-of-eaten-book.com for cooking & coaching tips!

Daily Meal Plan Menu

Week 8/ Day 51

Your Breakfast/Brunch Menu for today is:
1) Scrambled Egg - 2
2) Avocado - 1 Whole
3) Broccoli (Boil) - 1 Cup
4) Kale Salad (Stir-fry) - 1 Cup
5) Water & Lemon - 8 oz.
6) Probiotics - Once A Day
7) Vitamin B Complex
Estimated Calories: 320
Estimated Carbs: 11
Estimated Sugar: 1
Blood Pressure (Optional):
Cooking Tip: Use coconut oil to stir-fry kale for 2 minutes.

Your Dinner Menu for today is:
1) 100% Organic Grass-Fed Beef Burger - 1
2) Asparagus (Boil) - 8 Stalks
3) Broccoli (Boil) - 1 Cup
4) Slaw - 3 Tbsp
5) Water & Lemon - 8 oz.
Estimated Calories: 310
Estimated Carbs: 8
Estimated Sugar: 2
Blood Pressure (Optional):
Cooking Tip: Boil broccoli and asparagus separately.

Go to: the-garden-of-eaten-book.com for cooking & coaching tips!

Daily Meal Plan Menu

Week 8/ Day 52

Your Breakfast/Brunch Menu for today is:
1) Boiled Eggs - 2
2) Asparagus (Boil) - 8 Stalks
3) Broccoli (Boil) - 1 Cup
4) Waffle - 1/4 Serving
5) Water & Lemon - 8 oz.
6) Probiotics - Once A Day
7) Vitamin B Complex
Estimated Calories: 310
Estimated Carbs: 11.5
Estimated Sugar: 4
Blood Pressure (Optional):
Cooking Tip: Eggs can also scrambled or cooked sunny-side up.

Your Dinner Menu for today is:
1) 100% Organic Grass-Fed Beef Burger (Fiesta Bowl) - 1 (4 oz.)
2) Kale Salad (Stir-fry) - 1 Cup
3) Arugula Salad (Stir-fry) - 1 Cup
4) Black Beans - 3 Tbsp
5) Sour Cream - 2 Tbsp
6) Grain-Free Tortilla Chips (with *Lime*) - 5
7) Water & Lemon - 8 oz.
Estimated Calories: 480
Estimated Carbs: 23.5
Estimated Sugar: 1
Blood Pressure (Optional):
Cooking Tip: Mix cooked ground beef with black beans, sour cream & grain-free tortilla chips.

Go to: the-garden-of-eaten-book.com for cooking & coaching tips!

Daily Meal Plan Menu

Week 8/ Day 53

Your Breakfast/Brunch Menu for today is:
1) Sugar-Free Bacon - 2
2) Scrambled Eggs - 2
3) Kale Salad (Stir-fry) - 1 Cup
4) Arugula Salad (Stir-fry) - 1 Cup
5) Water & Lemon - 8 oz.
6) Probiotics - Once A Day
7) Vitamin B Complex
Estimated Calories: 320
Estimated Carbs: 7
Estimated Sugar: 0
Blood Pressure (Optional):
Cooking Tip: Use coconut oil to stir-fry kale & arugula for 2 minutes.

Your Dinner Menu for today is:
1) Scrambled Eggs - 2
2) Asparagus (Boil) - 8 Stalks
3) Broccoli (Boil) - 1 Cup
4) Kale Salad (Stir-fry) - 1 Cup
5) Slaw - 3 Tbsp
6) Water & Lemon - 8 oz.
Estimated Calories: 260
Estimated Carbs: 13.5
Estimated Sugar: 2
Blood Pressure (Optional):
Cooking Tip: Boil asparagus and broccoli separately.

Go to: the-garden-of-eaten-book.com for cooking & coaching tips!

Daily Meal Plan Menu

Week 8/ Day 54

Your Breakfast/Brunch Menu for today is:
1) Sausage Patty - 1
2) Scrambled Eggs - 2
3) Asparagus (Boil) - 8 Stalks
4) Broccoli (Boil) - 1 Cup
5) Water & Lemon - 8 oz.
6) Probiotics - Once A Day
7) Vitamin B Complex
Estimated Calories: 310
Estimated Carbs: 6
Estimated Sugar: 1
Blood Pressure (Optional):
Cooking Tip: Boil broccoli & asparagus separately.

Your Dinner Menu for today is:
1) Home Style Meatballs - 4
2) Broccoli (Boil) - 1 Cup
3) Black Beans - 3 Tbsp
4) Slaw - 3 Tbsp
5) Water & Lemon - 8 oz.
Estimated Calories: 310
Estimated Carbs: 11.5
Estimated Sugar: 3
Blood Pressure (Optional):
Cooking Tip: Mix slaw with avocado mayonnaise.

Go to: the-garden-of-eaten-book.com for cooking & coaching tips!

Daily Meal Plan Menu

Week 8/ Day 55

Your Breakfast/Brunch Menu for today is:
1) Sausage Patty - 1
2) Asparagus (Boil) - 8 Stalks
3) Avocado - 1 Whole
4) Black Beans - 3 Tbsp
5) Slaw - 3 Tbsp
6) Water & Lemon - 8 oz.
7) Probiotics - Once A Day
8) Vitamin B Complex
Estimated Calories: 370
Estimated Carbs: 11.5
Estimated Sugar: 2
Blood Pressure (Optional):
Cooking Tip: Mix slaw with avocado oil mayonnaise.

Your Dinner Menu for today is:
1) Baked Marinated Chicken - 1
2) Broccoli (Boil) - 1 Cup
3) Asparagus (Boil) - 8 Stalks
4) Slaw - 3 Tbsp
5) Water & Lemon - 8 oz.
Estimated Calories: 210
Estimated Carbs: 8
Estimated Sugar: 2
Blood Pressure (Optional):
Cooking Tip: Boil broccoli and asparagus separately.

Go to: the-garden-of-eaten-book.com for cooking & coaching tips!

Daily Meal Plan Menu

Week 8/ Day 56

Your Breakfast/Brunch Menu for today is:
1) Sugar-Free Bacon - 2
2) Scrambled Egg - 2
3) Broccoli (Boil) - 1 Cup
4) Asparagus (Boil) - 8 Stalks
5) Waffle - 1/4 Serving
6) Water & Lemon - 8 oz.
7) Probiotics - Once A Day
8) Vitamin B Complex
Estimated Calories: 370
Estimated Carbs: 11.5
Estimated Sugar: 4
Blood Pressure (Optional):
Cooking Tip: Boil broccoli and asparagus separately.

Your Dinner Menu for today is:
1) Turkey Burger - 1
2) Kale Salad (Stir-fry) - 1 Cup
3) Arugula Salad (Stir-fry) - 1 Cup
4) Black Beans - 3 Tbsp
5) Sour Cream - 2 Tsp
6) Slaw - 3 Tbsp
7) Water & Lemon - 8 oz.
Estimated Calories: 310
Estimated Carbs: 16.5
Estimated Sugar: 2
Blood Pressure (Optional):
Cooking Tip: Use coconut oil to stir-fry kale and arugula salad.

Go to: the-garden-of-eaten-book.com for cooking & coaching tips!

GROCERY LIST
(Approved & Organic)

- Organic Avocados
- Organic Fresh Slaw
- Organic Fresh Cabbage
- Organic Fresh Asparagus
- Organic Fresh Kale Salad
- Organic Fresh Cauliflower
- Organic Fresh Arugula Salad
- Organic Black Beans (*Eden* Brand only)
- Organic Premium Broccoli Florets (*Cascadian Farm* Brand)
- Organic Ghee Clarified Butter with Himalayan Pink Salt (100% Grass Fed)
- Avocado Cooking Spray (*Chosen* Brand)
- Mayonnaise with Avocado Oil (*Primal Kitchen* Brand)
- Celtic Sea Salt Fine Ground
- Organic Pepper
- Organic Coconut Oil
- Organic Garlic Sea Salt
- Organic Vitamin B (*Garden of Life* Brand)
- Organic Probiotics (*Garden of Life* Brand)
- Grain-Free Tortilla Chips (*Siete* Brand)
- Grain-Free Gluten Free Paleo Waffles (*Liberate Specialty Food* Brand)
- Turkey Bacon (*Applegate Organics* Brand)
- Organic Turkey Burgers (*Applegate Organics* Brand)
- All Natural Fully Cooked Original Pork Sausage Patties (*Wellshire* Brand)
- Organic Applewood Smoked Sugar-Free Uncured Bacon (*North Country Smoke House* Brand)
- 100% Boneless Skinless Organic Chicken Breasts (*Whole Foods* Brand)
- 100% Boneless Skinless Organic Chicken Thighs (*Whole Foods* Brand)
- 100% Boneless Skinless Organic Chicken Wings (*Whole Foods* Brand)

100% Organic Beef Grass-Fed Burger (*The Organic Meat Co.* Brand)
100% Grass-Fed Beef Homestyle Meatball (*Cooked Perfect* Brand)
Organic Pasture Raised Eggs/Non-GMO (*Vital Farms* Brand)
Organic Volcano Lemon Burst Juice
Spring Water (BPA-Free or glass bottle)
Mountain Valley Spring Water (BPA-Free or glass bottle)
Alkaline Water (BPA-Free or glass bottle) for up to 3 or 4 weeks

APPROVED FOOD SUBSTITUTE LIST

Approved Meats:
Organic Sugar-Free Bacon (*North Country Smoke House* Brand)
Organic Turkey Bacon (*Applegate Organics* Brand)
Organic Canadian Bacon (*Applegate Organics* Brand)
Organic Skinless Chicken Breast (*Whole Foods* Brand)
Organic Skinless Chicken Thighs (*Whole Foods* Brand)
Organic Turkey Burger (*Applegate Organics* Brand)
100% Organic Grass-Fed Beef Burger (*The Organic Meat Co.* Brand)
Organic Homestyle Beef Meatballs (*Cooked Perfect* Brand)
Wild Caught Salmon
Wild Caught Shrimp
Wild Caught Cod Fish
Wild Caught Sardines
(All meat must be baked or grilled)

Approved Vegetables
Organic Broccoli
Organic Bok Choy
Organic Fresh Slaw
Organic Kale Salad
Organic Fresh *Garlic*
Organic Fresh Onions
Organic Swiss Chard
Organic Butter Lettuce
Organic Cauliflower
Organic Arugula Salad
Organic Fresh Cabbage
Organic Collard Greens
Organic Mustard Greens
Organic Fresh Asparagus
Organic Romaine Lettuce
Organic Fresh Brussel Sprouts
Organic Black Beans (*Eden* Brand Only)

Approved Fruit
Avocado

Approved Oils
Organic Coconut Oil
Organic Extra Virgin Olive Oil
Organic Avocado Oil (*Chosen* Brand)

Approved Condiments:
Organic Sour Cream
Organic Ranch Dressing (*Primal Kitchen* Brand)
Organic Italian Dressing (*Primal Kitchen* Brand)
Organic Avocado Oil Mayonnaise (*Primal Kitchen* Brand)

Approved Spices
Organic Pepper
Organic Celtic Salt
Organic Garlic Salt
Organic Seasoning Salt

Approved Drinks:
Mountain Valley Spring Water (Glass bottle or BPA-Free)
Alkaline Water in a BPA-Free Bottle (For up to 3 or 4 weeks)

www.ingramcontent.com/pod-product-compliance
Lightning Source LLC
Chambersburg PA
CBHW070338230426
43663CB00011B/2364